I0758595

The Role of Nutrition in Osteomyelitis Healing and Prevention

The Role of Nutrition in Osteomyelitis Healing and Prevention

Latest Insights and Recommendations

Victor Asher

Other Books by Victor Asher

Simple Exercise for Osteoporosis

Achieving & Maintaining a Healthy Life

The Inevitable Journey of Grief

Understanding the Quality & Benefits of a Revitalizing Sleep

A Step – By – Step Guide for Dads

Optimizing Life with Osteoarthritis

Unveiling The Hidden Benefits Of Walking And Hiking

Relationship's Hurricanes

Eating For Health

Cook well Eat well and live well

Exercise and Prostate Health

The Enigmatic African Grey Parrot

Understanding & Taming the Fiery Nature of Anger

How to Achieve Financial Stability in Today's World

Coping with Adolescence

Alternative and Complementary Therapies for Rheumatoid Arthritis

The Path to Success

Life Changing Quotes on Pages

Imaginative Tales to Dream Away

Beyond The Throne

60 Mind-loving Stories for Seniors

Dedication

This book is dedicated to God for His grace and wisdom, to my family, to my beautiful readers who will find this book relevant to them, and to everyone who has loved, supported, and encouraged me along the way. I would not be in the position I am in today without your unshakable faith in me. I dedicate this book to all my readers' especially those who are having issues with osteomyelitis and desire to be healthy as this will sincerely be of importance to you all.

Table of Contents

Acknowledgement

I want to sincerely thank God for providing the means and insight that guided me during the writing of this book. I cannot forget my family members, whose encouragement and support have given me bravery and motivation throughout the process.

Thank you to my editor and publisher for their crucial advice and help in bringing this project to its successful conclusion. I would like to express my gratitude to everyone who so kindly contributed their time and knowledge to this project and added their wisdom. I want to express my gratitude to my friends as well, I appreciate all of your steadfast love and support throughout the journey.

I like to thank stock.adobe.com and vinmec.com for those wonderful images, you all are wonderful.

Finally, I extend my thanks to each and every one of you for purchasing and reading my work. I am thankful it met your needs and added to your knowledge. I sincerely value each and every one of you and think you're all fantastic.

Introduction

In the realm of healthcare, the significance of proper nutrition cannot be understated. It serves as a cornerstone for maintaining optimal health and supporting the body's ability to combat various ailments. When it comes to a complex condition like osteomyelitis, where bone infection threatens the very foundation of our skeletal system, the role of nutrition takes on even greater importance.

Osteomyelitis, a severe infection of the bone, poses significant challenges in both its treatment and prevention. Traditionally, medical interventions such as antibiotics, surgical debridement, and long-term wound care have been the mainstays of combating this relentless adversary. However, emerging research has shed light on a critical aspect of osteomyelitis management that had long been overlooked: the role of nutrition.

Our understanding of the intricate interplay between nutrition and bone health has deepened in recent years, unveiling valuable insights into how diet and specific nutrients can influence the healing and prevention of osteomyelitis. By harnessing the power of proper nutrition, we may unlock a new frontier in our battle against this stubborn bone infection.

Imagine a scenario where nutrition acts as a shield, fortifying bones against invasion and accelerating the recovery process. Through an understanding of key nutrients, dietary interventions, and their effects on the immune system, healthcare professionals are gaining the power to bolster the body's defenses against osteomyelitis.

This book aims to delve into the latest scientific discoveries surrounding nutrition's impact on osteomyelitis. We will explore the key nutrients involved in bone health and how they can fortify the body's defense mechanisms against osteomyelitis. Additionally, we will discuss dietary recommendations and lifestyle modifications that can support the healing process and help prevent the recurrence of this debilitating condition.

From essential vitamins and minerals to the significance of macronutrients, we will explore the intricacies of the nutritional landscape in the context of osteomyelitis. Furthermore, we will examine the potential therapeutic implications of various dietary interventions and their ability to enhance the effectiveness of traditional treatments.

As we embark on this enlightening journey through the realm of nutrition and osteomyelitis, we hope to equip healthcare professionals and individuals alike with the knowledge needed to make informed decisions about their dietary choices, ultimately leading to improved outcomes and a stronger defense against this formidable bone infection.

So, let us delve into the latest insights and recommendations on the role of nutrition in osteomyelitis healing and prevention, unraveling the potential of food as a formidable ally in our fight against this challenging condition.

Chapter One

Osteomyelitis

Osteomyelitis is a serious and often painful infection of the bone. It occurs when bacteria or other infectious organisms invade the bone tissue, leading to inflammation, destruction of bone, and potential complications if left untreated. Osteomyelitis can affect any bone in the body, but it commonly occurs in the long bones of the arms and legs, the spine, and the pelvis.

About 2 to 5 people out of every 10,000 are affected by osteomyelitis. One of the first diseases ever known to man. More than 250 million years have been uncovered by scientists. People who smoke and those who suffer from long-term illnesses like diabetes or kidney failure are more likely to acquire osteomyelitis. If a diabetic person has foot ulcers, they run the risk of developing osteomyelitis.

The infection can occur through various routes, including:

1. **Hematogenous spread**

Bacteria from an existing infection elsewhere in the body, such as a urinary tract infection or respiratory infection, can enter the bloodstream and spread to the bone. Typically, *Staphylococcus aureus* is the cause of the blood infection, although it is possible that another bacterial or fungi species can also be responsible for example, *Streptococcus* species, *Escherichia coli, Pseudomonas aeruginosa*, and various fungi like *Candida* species

The specific microorganism involved may depend on factors such as the primary infection site, the individual's immune status, and other host-related factors.

2. Direct inoculation

This occurs when bacteria are introduced into the bone tissue through an open fracture, surgical procedure, or deep wound. Unlike contiguous spread, where the infection spreads from nearby soft tissues to the bone, direct inoculation bypasses the soft tissues and directly infects the bone.

3. Contiguous spread

Infections from nearby soft tissues, such as cellulitis or an abscess, can spread to the adjacent bone.

When there is an infection in the soft tissues, such as cellulitis (a bacterial skin infection) or an abscess (a collection of pus), the bacteria or other pathogens involved can extend their reach to the surrounding bone tissue.

The spread of infection from soft tissues to bone usually occurs when the infection is not effectively treated or if the immune system is compromised.

Signs and Symptoms

The signs and symptoms of osteomyelitis may vary depending on the duration and severity of the infection.

Common symptoms include:

- Localized pain and tenderness over the infected area.
- Swelling, redness, and warmth at the site of infection.
- Limited range of motion and difficulty using the affected limb.
- Fever, chills, and general malaise in cases of systemic infection.
- Open wounds or draining sinuses near the infected bone in chronic cases.

Risk Factors of Osteomyelitis

Several risk factors can increase a person's susceptibility to developing osteomyelitis. These risk factors can be categorized into different groups:

1. Pre-existing Medical Conditions

- **Diabetes**

Uncontrolled diabetes can impair blood circulation and weaken the immune system, making individuals more vulnerable to infections, including osteomyelitis.

- **Peripheral Vascular Disease**

Conditions that affect blood flow to the extremities, such as peripheral arterial disease, can increase the risk of developing osteomyelitis due to compromised blood supply to the bones.

- **Immunodeficiency Disorders**

Conditions that weaken the immune system, such as HIV/AIDS, leukemia, or autoimmune disorders, can make individuals more susceptible to infections, including osteomyelitis.

- **Chronic Kidney Disease**

Kidney disease can impair the body's ability to fight off infections, increasing the risk of developing osteomyelitis.

2. Recent Trauma or Surgery

- **Open Fractures**

When a bone breaks and punctures the skin, it provides a direct pathway for bacteria to enter the bone, leading to infection.

- **Orthopedic Surgery**

Procedures involving joint replacements, fracture fixation, or spinal instrumentation carry a small risk of introducing bacteria into the bone, potentially leading to osteomyelitis.

3. Circulatory Disorders

- **Peripheral Arterial Disease**

Reduced blood flow to the extremities can impair the delivery of oxygen and nutrients to the bones, making them more susceptible to infection.

- **Venous Insufficiency**

Chronic venous insufficiency, characterized by poor blood flow in the veins, can contribute to tissue damage and increase the risk of developing osteomyelitis.

4. Compromised Immune System

- **Steroid Therapy**

Long-term or high-dose steroid use can suppress the immune system, making individuals more susceptible to infections.

- **Chemotherapy**

Cancer treatments, particularly chemotherapy, can weaken the immune system, making patients more prone to infections, including osteomyelitis.

5. Skin Infections and Ulcers

- **Cellulitis**

Bacterial skin infections, such as cellulitis, can spread to the underlying bones, leading to osteomyelitis.

- **Pressure Ulcers**

Open wounds, such as pressure ulcers or bedsores, provide an entry point for bacteria to infect the bone.

6. Intravenous Drug Use

- Injecting drugs intravenously can introduce bacteria directly into the bloodstream, increasing the risk of developing osteomyelitis.

It's important to note that while these risk factors can increase the likelihood of developing osteomyelitis, not everyone with these factors will necessarily develop the condition. Maintaining good overall health, practicing proper wound care, and managing underlying medical conditions can help reduce the risk of osteomyelitis.

Diagnosis

Osteomyelitis is a serious infection of the bone, typically caused by bacteria. It can be challenging to diagnose as the symptoms can be similar to other conditions, and various diagnostic tests may be needed to confirm the presence of osteomyelitis.

Here are some common methods used for diagnosing osteomyelitis:

1. Medical history and physical examination

The doctor will ask about your symptoms, medical history, and any recent injuries or surgeries. They will also perform a physical examination to assess the affected area, looking for signs of inflammation, tenderness, or swelling.

2. Blood tests

Blood tests can help identify signs of infection, such as an elevated white blood cell count (WBC), increased erythrocyte sedimentation rate (ESR), and C-reactive protein (CRP) levels. These markers indicate the presence of inflammation in the body.

3. Imaging studies

Different imaging techniques may be used to visualize the affected bone and surrounding tissues. These include:

- X-rays: X-rays can detect changes in the bone, such as bone destruction, periosteal reaction (new bone formation around the affected area), or sequestra (dead bone fragments).
- Magnetic Resonance Imaging (MRI): MRI provides detailed images of bones, soft tissues, and infections. It can help identify early signs of osteomyelitis, detect the extent of the infection, and assess the surrounding soft tissues.
- Computed Tomography (CT) scan: CT scans may be used to provide more detailed images of the bone and surrounding structures. They can help evaluate the extent of bone destruction and identify any associated abscesses or soft tissue involvement.

4. Bone biopsy

A bone biopsy is the most definitive diagnostic test for osteomyelitis. It involves taking a small sample of bone tissue from the affected area for laboratory analysis. The sample is cultured to identify the specific bacteria causing the infection and determine the most effective antibiotic treatment.

It's important to note that the diagnostic process may vary depending on the individual case, and additional tests or procedures may be required based on the specific circumstances and the doctor's judgment. It is essential to consult with a healthcare professional for an accurate diagnosis and appropriate treatment plan.

If left untreated, osteomyelitis can lead to severe complications, such as the formation of abscesses, bone death (called sequestrum), pathological fractures, joint destruction, and the spread of infection to surrounding tissues.

Early diagnosis, prompt treatment, and appropriate management of osteomyelitis are crucial for improving outcomes and reducing the risk of long-term complications.

Chapter Two

Nutrition and Osteomyelitis

Osteomyelitis, a formidable infection of the bone, demands a multifaceted approach to treatment and prevention. While antibiotics and surgical interventions play a crucial role in combating this relentless condition, the impact of nutrition should not be underestimated. Emerging research is shedding light on the pivotal role that nutrition plays in both healing and preventing osteomyelitis.

Proper nutrition serves as a vital ally in bolstering the body's immune response, facilitating bone healing, and reducing the risk of infection recurrence. Essential nutrients, such as vitamins, minerals, and macronutrients, work in harmony to support the intricate processes involved in bone health and immunity.

Vitamin D, often referred to as the "sunshine vitamin," is receiving significant attention in the context of osteomyelitis. This essential vitamin not only plays a crucial role in bone health and calcium absorption but also possesses potent immunomodulatory properties. Adequate vitamin D levels have been associated with a decreased risk of osteomyelitis and enhanced healing outcomes.

Another key player in the nutritional arsenal against osteomyelitis is vitamin C. Known for its antioxidant properties and its role in collagen synthesis, vitamin C is vital for wound healing and tissue repair. Studies have shown that vitamin C deficiency can impair the body's ability to fight infections, including osteomyelitis.

Additionally, a balanced intake of macronutrients, such as proteins, carbohydrates, and fats, is essential for supporting the body's immune response and providing the energy needed for optimal healing. Proteins, in particular, play a critical role in tissue repair and immune function. Adequate protein intake is crucial for the formation of new bone tissue and the prevention of muscle wasting, which can be detrimental to overall recovery.

Moreover, maintaining a well-rounded diet that includes a variety of fruits, vegetables, whole grains, and lean sources of protein can supply the body with a wide array of vitamins, minerals, and phytonutrients. These compounds act synergistically to support immune function, reduce inflammation, and promote overall health, thereby enhancing the body's ability to combat infections like osteomyelitis.

While nutrition alone cannot eradicate osteomyelitis, it serves as a powerful adjunct to conventional treatments. By optimizing nutritional intake, healthcare providers can provide patients with the tools necessary to support their immune systems, promote bone healing, and reduce the risk of future infections.

In the quest to conquer osteomyelitis, a comprehensive approach that recognizes the pivotal role of nutrition is essential. By integrating the latest insights and recommendations on nutrition into treatment plans, healthcare professionals and patients can harness the power of nourishment to strengthen the body's defenses, expedite healing, and pave the way towards a brighter, healthier future.

Nutritional Requirements for Osteomyelitis Healing

When it comes to osteomyelitis healing, proper nutrition plays a critical role in supporting the body's immune response, promoting tissue repair, and enhancing overall recovery.

Here are some key nutritional requirements that are important for individuals with osteomyelitis:

1. Protein

Adequate protein intake is crucial for healing and repairing damaged tissues, including bones. Protein provides the building blocks necessary for tissue regeneration and supports the immune system. Good sources of protein include lean meats, poultry, fish, eggs, dairy products, legumes, and plant-based protein sources like tofu and quinoa.

2. Vitamin C

Vitamin C is essential for collagen synthesis, a protein that plays a key role in wound healing and tissue repair. It also has antioxidant properties that help reduce inflammation. Citrus fruits, berries, kiwi, peppers, broccoli, and leafy green vegetables are excellent sources of vitamin C.

3. Vitamin D

Vitamin D is important for bone health as it aids in calcium absorption. It also possesses immunomodulatory properties, which can be beneficial in fighting infections like osteomyelitis. Natural sources of vitamin D include sunlight exposure and foods like fatty fish (salmon, mackerel), egg yolks, fortified dairy products, and fortified plant-based milk alternatives.

4. Calcium and Phosphorus

These minerals are essential for maintaining bone health and promoting bone healing. Good sources of calcium include dairy products, leafy green vegetables, fortified plant-based milk alternatives, and certain fish like sardines. Phosphorus can be obtained from foods such as dairy products, meat, fish, poultry, nuts, and legumes.

5. Omega-3 Fatty Acids

Omega-3 fatty acids have anti-inflammatory properties and can help reduce inflammation associated with osteomyelitis. Good sources of omega-3 fatty acids include fatty fish (salmon, mackerel, sardines), walnuts, flaxseeds, and chia seeds.

6. Antioxidants

Including a variety of fruits and vegetables in the diet provides a rich supply of antioxidants. Antioxidants help reduce oxidative stress and inflammation, supporting the healing process. Berries, leafy greens, tomatoes, carrots, and bell peppers are examples of antioxidant-rich foods.

7. Hydration

Staying hydrated is important for overall health and supports proper circulation, which aids in delivering essential nutrients to the affected areas. Water is the best choice for hydration, but herbal teas and natural fruit juices (without added sugars) can also contribute to fluid intake.

It's worth noting that individual nutritional needs may vary depending on factors such as age, overall health, and any underlying medical conditions. Consulting with a healthcare professional or registered dietitian can help tailor a nutrition plan specific to an individual's needs and optimize the healing process in the context of osteomyelitis.

Essential nutrients for bone health: Calcium, vitamin D, and phosphorus

Bone health is influenced by several essential nutrients, with calcium, vitamin D, and phosphorus playing key roles in maintaining strong and healthy bones.

Here's an overview of how these nutrients contribute to bone health:

1. Calcium

Calcium is the primary mineral responsible for the strength and density of bones. It provides the structural framework that supports the body and helps to resist fractures. Calcium is continuously deposited and withdrawn from bones in a process called remodeling, which helps maintain bone integrity. Adequate calcium intake is essential throughout life, particularly during periods of rapid growth (such as childhood and adolescence) and for the prevention of age-related bone loss. Good dietary sources of calcium include dairy products, leafy green vegetables, fortified plant-based milk, and calcium-rich seafood like sardines.

2. Vitamin D

Vitamin D is necessary for optimal calcium absorption and utilization. It helps regulate the levels of calcium and phosphorus in the body, which are essential for bone mineralization. Without adequate vitamin D, the body struggles to absorb sufficient calcium from the diet, leading to reduced bone mineral density and an increased risk of fractures. Vitamin D can be synthesized in the skin when exposed to sunlight and can also be obtained from dietary sources such as fatty fish (e.g., salmon, mackerel), fortified dairy products, and egg yolks. In some cases, supplementation may be recommended, especially in individuals with limited sun exposure or certain medical conditions.

3. Phosphorus

Phosphorus is another mineral that contributes to bone health. It works in conjunction with calcium to form hydroxyapatite crystals, which provide strength and rigidity to bones. Adequate phosphorus intake is important for maintaining the mineral balance in bones. Phosphorus is found in a variety of foods, including dairy products, meat, poultry, fish, nuts, and legumes.

It's worth noting that other nutrients also play a role in bone health. For example, vitamin K, magnesium, and various trace minerals like zinc and copper are involved in bone formation and remodeling processes. Additionally, a well-balanced diet that includes a variety of nutrient-rich foods is important for overall bone health and overall health.

If you have specific concerns about bone health or nutritional needs, it's advisable to consult with a healthcare professional or a registered dietitian who can provide personalized guidance based on your individual circumstances.

Protein for tissue repair: Role of adequate protein intake in enhancing healing processes

Adequate protein intake plays a crucial role in enhancing healing processes, particularly tissue repair. Proteins are the building blocks of the body and are essential for the growth, maintenance, and repair of tissues. When it comes to wound healing and tissue repair, here's how protein intake influences these processes:

1. Collagen synthesis

Collagen is a major component of connective tissues, including skin, tendons, ligaments, and blood vessels. It provides strength and structure to these tissues. Protein is necessary for the synthesis of collagen, as collagen molecules are made up of amino acids derived from dietary protein sources. Adequate protein intake ensures the availability of essential amino acids needed for collagen synthesis, supporting the formation of strong and healthy new tissue during the healing process.

2. Cell growth and proliferation

Protein is essential for cell growth, replication, and the production of new cells during tissue repair. When a wound occurs, the body needs to generate new cells to replace the damaged ones. Proteins provide the necessary amino acids for cell growth and division, supporting the proliferation of cells involved in wound healing, such as fibroblasts and keratinocytes.

3. Immune function

Protein is vital for a healthy immune system, which is crucial for efficient wound healing. During the healing process, the immune system helps fight off potential infections and supports tissue repair.

Antibodies, cytokines, and other immune molecules involved in the immune response are protein-based. Adequate protein intake supports the production of these immune components, enhancing the body's ability to combat infections and promote healing.

4. Enzyme production and function

Many enzymes involved in wound healing are protein-based. These enzymes facilitate various biochemical reactions necessary for tissue repair, such as the breakdown of damaged tissue, the synthesis of new tissue components, and the regulation of inflammation. Sufficient protein intake supports the production and activity of these enzymes, aiding in the healing process.

To ensure adequate protein intake for tissue repair and wound healing, it is generally recommended to consume a diet that includes a variety of protein sources. Good sources of protein include lean meats, poultry, fish, dairy products, eggs, legumes, nuts, and seeds. The exact protein requirements may vary depending on factors such as age, sex, overall health status, and the extent of the injury or wound. Consulting with a healthcare professional or a registered dietitian can provide personalized guidance on protein intake and overall nutritional needs during the healing process.

Micronutrients: Vitamin C, zinc, and iron as critical components in collagen synthesis and wound healing

Micronutrients such as vitamin C, zinc, and iron are indeed critical components in collagen synthesis and wound healing. Here's how each of these micronutrients contributes to these processes:

- **Vitamin C**

Vitamin C is an essential nutrient required for the synthesis of collagen, a protein that forms the structural framework of connective tissues, including skin, tendons, and blood vessels. Collagen is crucial for wound healing as it provides strength and integrity to the newly formed tissue. Vitamin C plays a key role in several steps of collagen synthesis, including the hydroxylation of proline and lysine amino acids, which is necessary for collagen's stability and cross-linking. Adequate vitamin C levels are necessary for proper wound healing and the formation of strong, healthy scar tissue.

- **Zinc**

Zinc is a micronutrient that is involved in various physiological processes, including collagen synthesis and immune function. It plays a critical role in the proliferation of cells involved in wound healing, such as fibroblasts and keratinocytes. Zinc is also necessary for the activity of enzymes involved in collagen synthesis, such as collagenase and elastase. Additionally, zinc is involved in immune function and helps protect against infections, which can hinder the wound healing process. Adequate zinc levels are essential for proper wound healing and tissue repair.

- **Iron**

Iron is a mineral that is essential for oxygen transport and plays a crucial role in various cellular processes. In wound healing, iron is necessary for the formation of new blood vessels (angiogenesis) and the oxygenation of tissues, which is vital for cell growth and collagen synthesis. Iron is also involved in immune function and the defense against infections.

Adequate iron levels are necessary for optimal wound healing and to support the body's energy requirements during the healing process.

It's important to note that while vitamin C, zinc, and iron are important for wound healing, they should be obtained through a balanced diet or, in some cases, under the guidance of a healthcare professional. If you have specific concerns about wound healing or micronutrient deficiencies, it's advisable to consult with a healthcare professional who can provide personalized advice and guidance.

Additionally, it's worth mentioning that wound healing is a complex process that involves various factors beyond these micronutrients, including other vitamins, minerals, proteins, and the overall nutritional status of an individual. A well-balanced diet that includes a variety of nutrient-rich foods is crucial for supporting optimal wound healing and overall health.

Omega-3 fatty acids: Potential anti-inflammatory effects and their influence on immune response

Omega-3 fatty acids are a type of polyunsaturated fatty acids that are considered essential nutrients because they are necessary for maintaining overall health and cannot be synthesized by the human body. They are primarily found in fatty fish (such as salmon, tuna, and mackerel), as well as in certain plant sources like flaxseeds, chia seeds, and walnuts.

Omega-3 fatty acids, particularly eicosapentaenoic acid (EPA) and docosahexaenoic acid (DHA), have been extensively studied for their potential anti-inflammatory effects and their influence on the immune response. Here's how they contribute to these processes:

- **Anti-inflammatory effects**

Omega-3 fatty acids have been shown to modulate the body's inflammatory response. They can inhibit the production of pro-inflammatory molecules, such as cytokines and prostaglandins, thereby reducing inflammation. By promoting a balanced immune response and decreasing excessive inflammation, omega-3 fatty acids may help mitigate chronic inflammatory conditions like rheumatoid arthritis, inflammatory bowel disease, and certain skin conditions.

- **Immune system modulation**

Omega-3 fatty acids play a role in regulating immune cell function. They can affect the activity of various immune cells, including macrophages, B cells, and T cells. These fatty acids may help enhance the body's defense against infections by improving immune cell communication and supporting their optimal functioning. They may also help in regulating autoimmune responses, where the immune system mistakenly attacks healthy cells.

- **Resolution of inflammation**

In addition to reducing inflammation, omega-3 fatty acids are involved in the resolution of inflammation. They promote the production of specialized pro-resolving mediators (SPMs), such as resolvins and protectins, which actively work to dampen and resolve the inflammatory response. By promoting timely and effective resolution of inflammation, omega-3 fatty acids support tissue healing and prevent the development of chronic inflammatory conditions.

- **Maintaining cell membrane integrity**

Omega-3 fatty acids are incorporated into cell membranes and influence their fluidity and stability. This can impact the functioning of immune cells, as well as their ability to communicate and respond to inflammatory signals. By maintaining healthy cell membranes, omega-3 fatty acids support optimal immune cell activity and responsiveness.

It's worth noting that the balance between omega-3 and omega-6 fatty acids in the diet is crucial. Omega-6 fatty acids, found in vegetable oils and processed foods, can promote inflammation when consumed in excess. Therefore, achieving a proper ratio of omega-3 to omega-6 fatty acids is important for optimal health and immune function.

While omega-3 fatty acids show promise in promoting anti-inflammatory effects and modulating the immune response, it's important to remember that they are not a standalone treatment for medical conditions. They should be considered as part of a balanced diet and a comprehensive approach to healthcare. If you have specific health concerns or conditions, it's advisable to consult with a healthcare professional for personalized advice.

Antioxidants: Role in reducing oxidative stress and promoting healing

Antioxidants play a crucial role in reducing oxidative stress and promoting healing in the body. Oxidative stress occurs when there is an imbalance between the production of reactive oxygen species (ROS) and the body's ability to neutralize and eliminate them. ROS are highly reactive molecules that can cause damage to cells, proteins, and DNA if their levels become excessive.

Here are some ways in which antioxidants contribute to reducing oxidative stress and promoting healing:

- **Neutralizing free radicals**

Antioxidants can donate an electron to unstable free radicals, neutralizing their reactivity. This helps prevent the free radicals from causing damage to cellular structures. Common antioxidants include vitamins C and E, beta-carotene, and selenium.

- **Protecting against inflammation**

Oxidative stress can trigger inflammation in the body. Antioxidants can help reduce inflammation by inhibiting the production of pro-inflammatory molecules and modulating immune responses. This is important for promoting healing in conditions associated with inflammation, such as wounds or chronic diseases.

- **Supporting tissue repair**

Antioxidants are involved in the synthesis and repair of collagen, a protein essential for wound healing and maintaining the structural integrity of tissues. They also promote the growth and differentiation of cells involved in tissue regeneration.

- **Enhancing immune function**

Oxidative stress can weaken the immune system, making the body more susceptible to infections and impairing the healing process. Antioxidants help support immune function by protecting immune cells from oxidative damage and promoting their optimal function.

- **Improving blood flow and circulation**

Certain antioxidants, such as flavonoids found in fruits and vegetables, have been shown to improve blood flow and enhance vascular health. This can aid in delivering oxygen and nutrients to tissues, promoting healing and recovery.

- **Reducing chronic disease risk**

Chronic diseases such as cardiovascular disease, neurodegenerative disorders, and certain cancers are associated with oxidative stress. By reducing oxidative stress, antioxidants can help lower the risk of developing these conditions and promote overall health and well-being.

It's important to note that while antioxidants are beneficial, they are not a cure-all solution. A balanced diet rich in fruits, vegetables, whole grains, and healthy fats is the best way to obtain a variety of antioxidants. It's also important to consult with a healthcare professional before starting any antioxidant supplements, as excessive intake of certain antioxidants may have adverse effects.

Chapter Three

Optimizing Nutrition for Osteomyelitis Patients

In the battle against osteomyelitis, a comprehensive approach that incorporates optimal nutrition can significantly impact a patient's healing journey. Proper nourishment plays a vital role in supporting the immune system, facilitating tissue repair, and enhancing overall recovery. By understanding and implementing strategies to optimize nutrition for osteomyelitis patients, healthcare professionals can unlock the potential for improved outcomes and accelerated healing.

The complex interplay between nutrition and osteomyelitis is increasingly recognized as a critical component of comprehensive care. Through tailored dietary interventions, personalized supplementation, and a focus on essential nutrients, healthcare providers can harness the power of nutrition to strengthen the body's defenses and promote optimal healing.

This exploration of optimizing nutrition for osteomyelitis patients delves into the key considerations and strategies to ensure the delivery of vital nutrients that aid in combating infection, supporting tissue repair, and enhancing immune function. From adequate protein intake to the importance of specific vitamins and minerals, this journey uncovers the crucial role that nutrition plays in the multifaceted management of osteomyelitis.

By embracing a holistic approach that integrates the latest insights and individualized nutrition plans, healthcare professionals empower osteomyelitis patients to take an active role in their recovery. Together, they navigate the intricate realm of nutrition, leveraging its potential to expedite healing, reduce complications, and enhance overall well-being.

As we embark on this exploration of optimizing nutrition for osteomyelitis patients, we unlock the power of nourishment as a valuable ally in the fight against this challenging condition. Join us as we delve into the strategies, insights, and recommendations that pave the way towards improved outcomes and a brighter future for those affected by osteomyelitis.

Assessment of nutritional status: Screening tools and evaluations to identify nutritional deficiencies.

Assessing nutritional status is essential to identify potential nutritional deficiencies and develop appropriate interventions. Healthcare professionals employ various screening tools and evaluations to evaluate an individual's nutritional status.

Here are some commonly used methods:

1. Dietary Assessment

This involves analyzing an individual's dietary intake to determine the adequacy of nutrient consumption. It can be done through methods such as food diaries, 24-hour recalls, and food frequency questionnaires. Dietary assessments provide valuable insights into nutrient intake patterns and help identify potential deficiencies or excessive intake.

2. Anthropometric Measurements

Anthropometric measurements assess body composition and provide information about growth, muscle mass, and fat stores. Common measurements include height, weight, body mass index (BMI), waist circumference, and skinfold thickness. Comparing these measurements to standardized growth charts or reference values helps identify malnutrition, obesity, or other deviations from the norm.

3. Biochemical Analysis

Blood tests can assess various biomarkers that reflect nutritional status. Examples include serum albumin, prealbumin, transferrin, vitamin and mineral levels (e.g., vitamin D, iron, folate), and markers of inflammation (e.g., C-reactive protein). Abnormalities in these biomarkers can indicate nutritional deficiencies or underlying health conditions affecting nutrient metabolism.

4. Clinical Evaluation

Healthcare professionals may conduct a physical examination to assess signs and symptoms of malnutrition or specific nutrient deficiencies. This can include examining the skin, hair, nails, oral cavity, and muscle mass. Clinical indicators, such as the presence of edema or poor wound healing, can also provide insights into nutritional status.

5. Subjective Global Assessment (SGA)

SGA is a comprehensive method that combines clinical evaluation, dietary assessment, and medical history. It involves interviewing the individual and collecting information on weight changes, appetite, gastrointestinal symptoms, functional capacity, and disease-related factors. SGA categorizes individuals into well-nourished, moderately malnourished, or severely malnourished categories.

6. Malnutrition Screening Tools

Various screening tools are available to quickly identify individuals at risk of malnutrition. Examples include the Malnutrition Universal Screening Tool (MUST), Mini Nutritional Assessment (MNA), and Nutritional Risk Screening (NRS-2002). These tools incorporate multiple parameters such as weight loss, BMI, and acute disease to assess nutritional risk.

7. Functional Assessment

This type of assessment evaluates an individual's ability to perform daily activities and assesses their functional status. Impairments in functional abilities can be indicative of underlying malnutrition or inadequate nutrient intake.

8. Medical History and Clinical Indicators

A thorough medical history, including information about current and past medical conditions, surgeries, medications, and gastrointestinal issues, can provide important insights into nutritional status. Additionally, clinical indicators such as unintentional weight loss, poor appetite, fatigue, and impaired wound healing can suggest nutritional deficiencies.

It is important to note that these screening tools and evaluations provide a snapshot of an individual's nutritional status and may have limitations. A comprehensive assessment that combines multiple methods is often the most effective approach to identify nutritional deficiencies and develop appropriate interventions.

Interdisciplinary collaboration among healthcare professionals, including registered dietitians, is valuable in interpreting the findings and designing personalized nutrition plans to address specific nutritional needs. By utilizing these screening tools and evaluations, healthcare professionals can identify individuals at risk of nutritional deficiencies and tailor interventions to optimize their nutritional status, promoting overall health and well-being.

Individualized dietary plans: Tailoring nutritional interventions based on the patient's needs.

Individualized dietary plans play a crucial role in optimizing nutritional interventions for patients, as everyone has unique nutritional needs and requirements. Tailoring these interventions based on the patient's specific needs ensures that they receive the right balance of nutrients to support their health, promote healing, and prevent nutritional deficiencies.

Here are some key aspects of individualized dietary plans:

1. Nutrient Requirements

Individualized dietary plans consider the patient's age, sex, weight, height, activity level, and underlying medical conditions to determine their specific nutrient requirements. Factors such as increased protein intake for wound healing or higher calcium and vitamin D intake for bone health may be taken into account. Registered dietitians or healthcare professionals with expertise in nutrition can calculate and recommend appropriate nutrient targets.

2. Food Preferences and Allergies

Patient-centered dietary plans take into consideration the patient's food preferences, cultural background, and any dietary restrictions or allergies they may have. This helps ensure that the recommended foods and meals are acceptable and enjoyable for the individual, increasing their adherence to the plan.

3. Adequate Energy Intake

The energy needs of individuals vary based on factors such as age, weight, activity level, and overall health. Individualized dietary plans aim to provide an adequate amount of energy to support the patient's daily activities, metabolism, and healing process. This may involve adjusting portion sizes, meal frequency, and macronutrient distribution (carbohydrates, proteins, and fats) to meet energy requirements.

4. Nutrient-Dense Foods

Individualized dietary plans focus on incorporating nutrient-dense foods to meet the patient's nutritional needs. This includes a variety of fruits, vegetables, whole grains, lean proteins, and healthy fats. Emphasizing nutrient-dense foods ensures that the patient receives a wide range of vitamins, minerals, and antioxidants necessary for optimal health and healing.

5. Meal Timing and Frequency

Individualized plans may consider the patient's lifestyle and preferences when determining meal timing and frequency. Some patients may prefer three main meals with snacks in between, while others may prefer smaller, more frequent meals. The goal is to establish a meal pattern that suits the patient's schedule and allows for consistent nutrient intake throughout the day.

6. Education and Support

Individualized dietary plans should be accompanied by education and ongoing support from healthcare professionals or registered dietitians. This includes explaining the rationale behind the recommendations, providing meal planning guidance, addressing any concerns or questions, and monitoring progress. Regular follow-ups and adjustments to the plan may be necessary based on the patient's response and changing needs.

7. Nutritional Supplements

In some cases, individualized dietary plans may include the recommendation of specific nutritional supplements to address any identified deficiencies or to support the healing process. This may involve the use of oral supplements, such as vitamins, minerals, or specialized nutritional formulations, to ensure the patient's nutrient needs are met.

8. Monitoring and Evaluation

Regular monitoring and evaluation of the patient's progress are essential components of individualized dietary plans. This allows healthcare professionals to assess the effectiveness of the interventions, make any necessary adjustments, and address any challenges or concerns that may arise. Monitoring may involve regular weight checks, biochemical tests, or subjective assessments of the patient's well-being.

9. Long-term Lifestyle Changes

Individualized dietary plans aim to promote long-term lifestyle changes that support optimal nutrition beyond the immediate healing period. Education and support are provided to help patients make sustainable dietary choices and develop healthy eating habits that they can continue to follow even after their recovery.

10. Interdisciplinary Collaboration

Developing individualized dietary plans requires close collaboration between healthcare professionals, including registered dietitians, physicians, nurses, and other members of the healthcare team. By working together, they can ensure that the nutritional interventions align with the overall treatment plan and address the specific needs and goals of the patient.

By tailoring nutritional interventions based on the patient's needs, individualized dietary plans maximize the effectiveness of dietary interventions. They promote patient engagement, adherence, and overall satisfaction with the recommended nutrition plan. Collaboration between healthcare professionals and registered dietitians ensures that the patient's specific requirements are considered, leading to improved health outcomes and a better quality of life.

Importance of caloric sufficiency: Meeting energy requirements to support healing and prevent malnutrition.

Calorie sufficiency, or meeting the energy requirements of an individual, is of utmost importance in the context of osteomyelitis healing and prevention of malnutrition. Adequate calorie intake is necessary to support the body's physiological processes, promote tissue repair, and prevent muscle wasting. The energy derived from calories serves as the fuel for the body's healing mechanisms and is crucial for initiating and sustaining the healing process in individuals with osteomyelitis.

Insufficient calorie intake can have detrimental effects on the body, particularly in the context of osteomyelitis. One of the significant concerns is the preservation of lean body mass. When calorie intake is inadequate, the body may resort to breaking down its own muscle and organ tissues to meet its energy needs. This can lead to muscle wasting and compromised immune function, further hindering the healing process and increasing the risk of complications. By ensuring calorie sufficiency, individuals with osteomyelitis can help preserve their lean body mass and maintain optimal immune function.

Calorie sufficiency also plays a vital role in preventing malnutrition, a common concern among individuals with osteomyelitis. The condition itself can increase nutrient needs and impact appetite, making it even more crucial to meet energy requirements. Inadequate calorie intake can contribute to the development of malnutrition, which not only weakens the body's ability to heal but also increases the risk of infections and other complications. By providing sufficient calories, malnutrition can be prevented, leading to better outcomes for individuals with osteomyelitis.

Furthermore, adequate calorie intake supports immune function, which is crucial in managing and preventing infections associated with osteomyelitis. Insufficient energy intake can weaken the immune system, making individuals more susceptible to infections and impairing their ability to fight them off. By meeting energy needs through calorie sufficiency, individuals can support their immune function, enhance their body's defense mechanisms, and contribute to the effective management of osteomyelitis.

Calorie sufficiency also plays a role in enhancing nutrient absorption in the gastrointestinal tract. Some nutrients, such as fat-soluble vitamins, require sufficient calorie intake for proper absorption.

By meeting energy requirements, individuals can ensure that their bodies can effectively absorb and utilize essential nutrients, vitamins, and minerals necessary for optimal healing and overall nutritional status.

Meeting energy requirements through a well-balanced and nutrient-dense diet supports tissue repair, preserves lean body mass, strengthens the immune system, and enhances nutrient absorption. By ensuring adequate calorie intake, individuals can promote optimal healing, reduce the risk of complications, and support their overall well-being during the management of osteomyelitis.

Protein supplementation: Considerations for optimal protein intake and its impact on wound healing

Protein supplementation is a crucial component in optimizing protein intake and supporting wound healing in individuals with osteomyelitis. The healing process relies heavily on protein as it plays a vital role in tissue repair, collagen synthesis, and the formation of new cells. Considering the increased protein requirements in individuals with osteomyelitis, supplementation becomes essential to ensure adequate protein intake for optimal wound healing.

The quantity of protein is a key consideration when implementing protein supplementation. Determining the optimal protein intake depends on various factors such as age, weight, activity level, and the extent of tissue damage. Healthcare professionals, particularly registered dietitians, can assess the individual's protein needs and provide personalized recommendations. Generally, a protein intake ranging from 1.2 to 2 grams per kilogram of body weight per day is often recommended for individuals with wounds and infections.

Apart from quantity, the quality of protein is equally important. High-quality protein sources contain all the essential amino acids required for tissue repair and growth. Including lean meats, poultry, fish, eggs, dairy products, legumes, and soy products in the diet ensures a complete and balanced amino acid profile. Diversifying protein sources allows for a broader range of essential nutrients that support the wound healing process.

Timing and distribution of protein intake are critical considerations for optimal wound healing. Spreading protein intake evenly throughout the day ensures a continuous supply of amino acids for tissue repair. Incorporating protein-rich foods in each meal, such as lean meats, fish, eggs, or legumes, can effectively meet protein needs. Additionally, regular meals and snacks with protein-rich options should be emphasized to support the ongoing healing process.

In cases where meeting protein requirements through a regular diet alone is challenging, nutritional supplements can be beneficial. Protein supplements, such as whey protein, casein protein, or plant-based protein powders, offer convenient options to augment protein intake. These supplements can be easily mixed with liquids or added to foods, making them practical choices for individuals who may struggle to meet their protein needs through regular meals.

Consideration should be given to individuals with specific medical conditions that may affect protein metabolism or digestion. For instance, individuals with renal impairment may require specialized protein recommendations.

It is crucial to consult with healthcare professionals to ensure protein supplementation is tailored to individual needs and any specific medical considerations.

Monitoring wound healing progress, nutritional status, and protein intake is essential in optimizing protein supplementation. Regular assessments by healthcare professionals allow for evaluation of the impact of protein supplementation on wound healing and the overall recovery process. Based on these assessments, adjustments to the protein intake can be made if necessary.

By considering the quantity and quality of protein, timing and distribution of protein intake, and any specific medical considerations, individuals can enhance the healing process and promote optimal recovery. Regular monitoring and consultation with healthcare professionals ensure that protein supplementation is effective and aligned with individual needs.

Micronutrient supplementation: Addressing specific deficiencies to promote bone health and immune function.

Micronutrient supplementation is a crucial aspect of promoting bone health and immune function in individuals with osteomyelitis. Micronutrients, including vitamins and minerals, play essential roles in various physiological processes, such as bone formation, tissue repair, and immune response. Addressing specific deficiencies through targeted supplementation can provide the necessary micronutrients to support these processes and optimize healing outcomes.

Calcium and vitamin D are key micronutrients for bone health. Calcium is a vital component of bone structure, while vitamin D facilitates calcium absorption and utilization. Individuals with osteomyelitis may have increased calcium and vitamin D needs due to bone damage and potential malabsorption. Supplementation with calcium and vitamin D can help address deficiencies, promote bone healing, and support overall bone health.

Vitamin C is essential for collagen synthesis, a critical component of connective tissues, including bones. It also plays a role in wound healing and immune function. Individuals with osteomyelitis may benefit from vitamin C supplementation to support collagen formation, enhance tissue repair, and strengthen the immune response.

Zinc is an important micronutrient involved in bone metabolism and immune function. It supports collagen synthesis, cell growth, and differentiation. Zinc supplementation may be beneficial for individuals with osteomyelitis, as it can aid in tissue repair and promote a healthy immune response.

Vitamin A is necessary for bone growth, development, and remodeling. It also plays a role in immune function. Supplementation with vitamin A can help address deficiencies and support bone health and immune response in individuals with osteomyelitis.

Omega-3 fatty acids, primarily found in fish oil, have anti-inflammatory properties and can help reduce inflammation associated with osteomyelitis. They also support immune function and contribute to overall health. Supplementation with omega-3 fatty acids may help modulate the immune response and promote healing in individuals with osteomyelitis.

In some cases, a comprehensive multivitamin and mineral supplement may be appropriate to address multiple micronutrient deficiencies.

These supplements provide a balanced combination of vitamins and minerals, ensuring adequate intake of various nutrients necessary for bone health, tissue repair, and immune function.

It is important to emphasize that micronutrient supplementation should be done under the guidance of healthcare professionals, particularly registered dietitians or physicians. They can assess individual nutritional needs, determine appropriate dosages, and monitor the effectiveness of supplementation. Regular monitoring of micronutrient levels and individual response to supplementation is crucial to evaluate the effectiveness of interventions and make necessary adjustments.

Supplementation with calcium, vitamin D, vitamin C, zinc, vitamin A, and omega-3 fatty acids can optimize nutrient status, support tissue repair, reduce inflammation, and enhance the immune response. Working closely with healthcare professionals ensures personalized recommendations and effective monitoring to achieve optimal outcomes for individuals with osteomyelitis.

Chapter Four

Nutrition and Osteomyelitis Prevention

Osteomyelitis, a serious and potentially debilitating bone infection, requires comprehensive management strategies to promote healing and prevent recurrence. While medical interventions such as antibiotics and surgical procedures are crucial, the role of nutrition in osteomyelitis prevention should not be overlooked. Proper nutrition plays a vital role in supporting immune function, promoting bone health, and optimizing overall healing. In this context, understanding the impact of nutrition on osteomyelitis prevention can help healthcare professionals and individuals alike implement effective dietary strategies to reduce the risk of infection and enhance the body's ability to combat this condition.

Healthy diet and lifestyle: Promoting a balanced diet and weight management to reduce the risk of osteomyelitis.

Maintaining a healthy diet and lifestyle is essential in reducing the risk of osteomyelitis. A balanced diet that provides adequate nutrition can strengthen the immune system, promote bone health, and support overall well-being.

Here are key considerations for promoting a healthy diet and lifestyle to minimize the risk of osteomyelitis:

1. Balanced Nutrition

Consuming a variety of nutrient-dense foods is crucial for optimal health. Include a wide range of fruits, vegetables, whole grains, lean proteins, and healthy fats in your diet. These foods provide essential vitamins, minerals, antioxidants, and phytochemicals that support immune function and overall health.

2. Adequate Calcium and Vitamin D Intake

Calcium and vitamin D are vital for bone health. Incorporate calcium-rich foods such as dairy products, leafy greens, and fortified foods into your diet. Additionally, spend time outdoors to promote natural vitamin D synthesis or consider vitamin D supplementation if necessary.

3. Hydration

Staying properly hydrated is essential for maintaining overall health and supporting immune function. Aim to drink an adequate amount of water throughout the day and limit the consumption of sugary beverages.

4. Weight Management

Maintaining a healthy weight can reduce the risk of certain conditions, including osteomyelitis. Excess weight can put strain on the bones and increase the likelihood of injury or infection. Follow a balanced diet, engage in regular physical activity, and consult with a healthcare professional to manage weight effectively.

5. Regular Exercise

Engaging in regular physical activity supports overall health and strengthens the musculoskeletal system. Weight-bearing exercises, such as walking, jogging, or resistance training, can help maintain bone density and reduce the risk of fractures.

6. Smoking Cessation

Smoking has been linked to an increased risk of osteomyelitis due to its negative impact on the immune system and blood circulation. Quitting smoking is crucial in reducing the risk of various infections, including osteomyelitis.

7. Good Hygiene Practices

Practicing good hygiene, such as regular handwashing, proper wound care, and avoiding contact with contaminated surfaces, can reduce the risk of bacterial infections that may lead to osteomyelitis.

By adopting a healthy diet and lifestyle, individuals can promote their overall well-being and reduce the risk of osteomyelitis. It is important to consult with healthcare professionals or registered dietitians to personalize dietary recommendations and lifestyle modifications based on individual needs and considerations.

Immune system support: Nutritional strategies to enhance immune function and prevent infections

Maintaining a strong immune system is crucial for preventing infections and promoting overall health. One of the key strategies to support immune function is to consume a well-balanced diet that includes a variety of fruits and vegetables. These plant-based foods are rich in essential vitamins, minerals, and antioxidants that provide the necessary nutrients for optimal immune health. Aim for a colorful mix of produce, as different colors indicate different beneficial nutrients.

In addition to fruits and vegetables, it's important to consume adequate protein, as it is necessary for the production of immune cells and antibodies. Include lean sources of protein such as poultry, fish, beans, lentils, nuts, and seeds in your diet. These foods not only provide protein but also contain other important nutrients that support immune function.

Probiotics are another important component of immune system support. Probiotics are beneficial bacteria that help maintain a healthy balance of gut flora, which in turn strengthens the immune system. You can find probiotics in fermented foods like yogurt, kefir, sauerkraut, and kimchi. Alternatively, you can consider taking a probiotic supplement to ensure an adequate intake of these beneficial bacteria.

Certain vitamins and minerals play a crucial role in supporting immune function. Vitamin C, for example, is well-known for its immune-boosting properties. Include citrus fruits, berries, kiwi, bell peppers, broccoli, and leafy greens in your diet to ensure an adequate intake of vitamin C. Vitamin D is also important, as it helps regulate immune responses. Exposure to sunlight is the best natural source of vitamin D, but you can also find it in fatty fish, egg yolks, and fortified dairy products. In some cases, a vitamin D supplement may be necessary, especially if you have limited sun exposure.

Zinc is another essential mineral for immune function. It helps in the production and function of immune cells. Include zinc-rich foods like oysters, beef, poultry, beans, nuts, and whole grains in your diet to support immune health. Staying hydrated is also important for optimal immune function. Proper hydration helps maintain the health and function of all body systems, including the immune system. Drink plenty of water throughout the day to support your immune system.

On the other hand, it's important to limit the consumption of added sugars and processed foods. Excessive intake of these foods can impair immune function and lead to inflammation. Instead, focus on whole, unprocessed foods that provide essential nutrients to support your immune system. Additionally, practicing good hygiene habits, such as regular handwashing, getting vaccinated, and avoiding close contact with sick individuals, is crucial for preventing infections.

Remember that a healthy lifestyle is a key factor in supporting immune function. Regular exercise, adequate sleep, stress management, and avoiding smoking and excessive alcohol consumption all contribute to a strong immune system. It's always a good idea to consult with a healthcare professional or registered dietitian for personalized advice tailored to your specific needs. They can help you create a well-rounded plan to support your immune system and overall health.

Diabetic management: Controlling blood sugar levels to minimize the risk of osteomyelitis in diabetic patients.

Diabetic management plays a crucial role in minimizing the risk of complications such as osteomyelitis in diabetic patients. Osteomyelitis is a serious infection of the bone that can occur when high blood sugar levels and impaired circulation compromise the immune system's ability to fight off infections.

Here are some key strategies for controlling blood sugar levels and reducing the risk of osteomyelitis

8.   Consistent blood sugar monitoring

Regularly monitoring blood sugar levels is essential for diabetic management. It allows you to understand how your body responds to different foods, medications, and activities. Work with your healthcare team to establish target ranges for blood sugar levels and use the appropriate monitoring methods, such as glucose meters or continuous glucose monitoring devices.

9.   Medication management

If you have been prescribed medication for diabetes, follow your healthcare provider's instructions carefully. This may include taking oral medications or insulin injections to help regulate blood sugar levels. Adhering to the prescribed dosage and schedule is crucial for maintaining stable blood sugar control.

10. Healthy eating

Adopting a well-balanced and consistent meal plan is vital for managing diabetes and preventing complications like osteomyelitis. Focus on consuming nutrient-dense foods that are low in added sugars and refined carbohydrates. Emphasize lean proteins, whole grains, fruits, vegetables, and healthy fats. Consider working with a registered dietitian to create a personalized meal plan that meets your specific dietary needs.

11. Portion control

Pay attention to portion sizes to prevent spikes in blood sugar levels. Use measuring cups, food scales, or visual references to ensure you're eating appropriate portions of different food groups. This practice can help regulate blood sugar levels and maintain a healthy weight.

12. Regular physical activity

Engaging in regular exercise can have a positive impact on blood sugar control. It helps improve insulin sensitivity and promotes weight management. Choose activities you enjoy and aim for a combination of aerobic exercises (such as brisk walking, cycling, or swimming) and strength training. Consult your healthcare provider before starting any exercise regimen, especially if you have any underlying health conditions.

13. Proper foot care

Diabetic patients are at an increased risk of foot complications, including osteomyelitis. Take proper care of your feet by regularly inspecting them for cuts, sores, or infections. Keep your feet clean and dry, and wear comfortable, well-fitting shoes and socks. Seek prompt medical attention for any foot-related concerns or infections.

14. Regular medical check-ups

Regular visits to your healthcare provider are essential for managing diabetes effectively. These check-ups allow for monitoring blood sugar control, evaluating potential complications, and adjusting treatment plans as needed. Your healthcare provider may conduct additional tests or screenings to assess your overall health and identify any potential risk factors for osteomyelitis or other complications.

15. Quit smoking

If you smoke, it's essential to quit. Smoking can impair blood circulation and increase the risk of infections and complications in diabetic patients. Seek support from healthcare professionals or smoking cessation programs to help you quit successfully.

Remember, managing diabetes is a lifelong commitment that requires regular self-care and collaboration with your healthcare team. By controlling blood sugar levels, adopting a healthy lifestyle, and taking preventive measures, you can minimize the risk of complications like osteomyelitis and maintain your overall health and well-being.

Hydration: Importance of adequate fluid intake for overall health and wound healing.

Adequate fluid intake and hydration are crucial for overall health and play a significant role in wound healing.

Here are some key points highlighting the importance of hydration:

1. Optimal bodily functions

The human body relies on water for numerous essential functions. Water helps regulate body temperature, aids in digestion, transports nutrients, oxygen, and waste products, and lubricates joints. Proper hydration ensures that these functions can be performed efficiently, promoting overall health.

2. Wound healing

Hydration is particularly important for wound healing. Adequate fluid intake helps maintain optimal blood flow and circulation, delivering essential nutrients and oxygen to the wound site. It also facilitates the removal of waste products and toxins, promoting a favorable environment for the healing process.

3. Tissue regeneration

Hydration supports the formation of new tissues and cells. Water is essential for the production of collagen, a protein that provides structure and strength to the skin, tendons, and other connective tissues. Sufficient hydration helps ensure that the body has the necessary resources to repair and regenerate damaged tissues.

4. Prevention of dehydration

Dehydration occurs when the body loses more fluids than it takes in. It can lead to various complications, including reduced blood volume, impaired kidney function, electrolyte imbalances, and decreased immune function. In the context of wound healing, dehydration can hinder the healing process and increase the risk of complications such as infections.

5. Moist wound environment

Proper hydration helps maintain a moist wound environment, which is essential for optimal healing. A moist environment supports cell migration, facilitates the formation of new blood vessels (angiogenesis), and promotes the development of granulation tissue. It also prevents the wound from drying out and forming a scab, as scab formation can impede healing and increase the risk of scarring.

6. Prevention of skin breakdown

Hydration plays a role in maintaining skin integrity and preventing skin breakdown. Dry and dehydrated skin is more prone to damage, cracking, and infection. By staying adequately hydrated, you can help keep your skin healthy, supple, and less susceptible to wounds and ulcers.

7. Fluid balance

Proper hydration is essential for maintaining fluid balance in the body. When the body is well-hydrated, it can effectively regulate electrolyte levels, which are essential for nerve function, muscle contraction, and maintaining proper pH balance. Electrolyte imbalances can disrupt normal bodily functions and hinder the healing process.

To ensure adequate hydration, it is generally recommended to drink an appropriate amount of water throughout the day. The exact amount can vary depending on factors such as age, activity level, climate, and overall health. In addition to water, other hydrating beverages such as herbal teas, diluted fruit juices, and electrolyte-rich drinks can contribute to overall fluid intake. However, it's important to limit the consumption of sugary or caffeinated beverages, as they can have diuretic effects and may not be as hydrating as plain water.

It's worth noting that individual hydration needs may vary, so it's important to listen to your body's signals and adjust your fluid intake accordingly. If you have specific health concerns or are undergoing wound healing, consult with your healthcare provider for personalized recommendations on fluid intake and hydration strategies.

Role of probiotics: Exploring the potential benefits of probiotics in maintaining a healthy gut microbiome and preventing infections

Probiotics are living microorganisms that, when consumed in adequate amounts, provide health benefits to the host. They are primarily known for their role in maintaining a healthy gut microbiome and supporting digestive health. Here are some potential benefits of probiotics in relation to gut health and infection prevention:

1. Restoring and maintaining gut microbiome balance

The gut microbiome is a complex community of microorganisms that plays a crucial role in digestion, nutrient absorption, immune function, and overall health. Probiotics, such as certain strains of bacteria (e.g., *Lactobacillus* and *Bifidobacterium*) and yeast (e.g., *Saccharomyces boulardii*), can help restore and maintain a healthy balance of beneficial bacteria in the gut. They can help counteract the negative effects of factors like antibiotics, poor diet, and stress that may disrupt the microbiome.

2. Enhancing immune function

A significant portion of the immune system resides in the gut. Probiotics can modulate the immune response by promoting the production of antimicrobial peptides, strengthening the gut barrier function, and influencing the activity of immune cells. By supporting a healthy gut microbiome, probiotics can help regulate immune function, potentially reducing the risk of infections and promoting immune resilience.

3. Preventing gastrointestinal infections

Certain strains of probiotics have been shown to have antimicrobial properties, which can help inhibit the growth of harmful bacteria and prevent gastrointestinal infections. For example, probiotics may reduce the risk and severity of diarrhea caused by pathogens such as *Clostridium difficile*, *Escherichia coli,* and *Salmonella.*

4. Managing antibiotic-associated side effects

Antibiotics can disrupt the natural balance of bacteria in the gut, often leading to antibiotic-associated diarrhea and other gastrointestinal issues. Probiotics, when taken alongside antibiotics, can help prevent or alleviate these side effects by promoting the restoration of the gut microbiome.

5. Supporting digestive health

Probiotics can contribute to the maintenance of a healthy digestive system by aiding in the breakdown and absorption of nutrients, reducing symptoms of digestive disorders (e.g., irritable bowel syndrome and inflammatory bowel disease), and promoting regular bowel movements.

6. Potential respiratory and urinary tract benefits

Some research suggests that certain probiotic strains may have a positive impact on respiratory and urinary tract health. Probiotics may help reduce the incidence and duration of respiratory infections, such as the common cold and upper respiratory tract infections. In the case of urinary tract infections, specific probiotics may inhibit the growth of uropathogenic bacteria and support urinary tract health.

It's important to note that the effectiveness of probiotics can vary depending on the specific strains used, the dosage, and individual factors. Not all probiotics have the same effects, and more research is needed to better understand their mechanisms of action and identify the most beneficial strains for specific health conditions.

If you are considering incorporating probiotics into your routine, it's recommended to choose products that have been tested for quality and efficacy. Consult with a healthcare professional, such as a doctor or registered dietitian, to determine the most appropriate probiotic strains, dosage, and duration of use based on your specific health needs and medical history.

Chapter Five

Challenges and Considerations

Addressing the nutritional needs of osteomyelitis patients can be complex and challenging due to various factors that can impact dietary intake and compliance. Healthcare professionals must navigate these challenges and consider several important factors to optimize nutritional support and enhance patient outcomes. Understanding the challenges and considerations involved in managing the nutritional aspects of osteomyelitis is crucial for developing effective strategies and providing patient-centered care.

This chapter will discuss some of the common challenges and considerations healthcare professionals encounter when addressing the nutritional needs of osteomyelitis patients and provide insights into how these challenges can be overcome to ensure optimal nutritional support and adherence to dietary recommendations. By addressing these challenges and considerations, healthcare professionals can play a key role in promoting the healing process, minimizing complications, and supporting the overall well-being of osteomyelitis patients.

Nutritional assessment in osteomyelitis patients: Identifying barriers and overcoming challenges

Nutritional assessment plays a crucial role in identifying the nutritional status and needs of osteomyelitis patients. However, there can be several challenges and barriers in conducting a comprehensive nutritional assessment in this population. Here are some considerations for overcoming these challenges:

1. Barriers to food intake

Osteomyelitis patients may face barriers to food intake, such as reduced appetite, pain during eating, or difficulty chewing and swallowing. It's important to address these barriers by providing pain management strategies, modifying food textures as needed, and offering smaller, frequent meals that are more manageable for the individual.

2. Malnutrition screening

Implementing a malnutrition screening tool can help identify patients at risk of malnutrition. Tools such as the Malnutrition Universal Screening Tool (MUST) or the Subjective Global Assessment (SGA) can be used to assess the nutritional status of osteomyelitis patients. Healthcare professionals should be trained to administer and interpret these screening tools accurately.

3. Dietary history and food preferences

Gathering a detailed dietary history and taking into account individual food preferences and cultural considerations is essential. This information helps in understanding the patient's usual eating habits, identifying potential nutrient deficiencies, and designing a personalized nutrition plan that is acceptable and feasible for the individual.

4. Collaborative approach

Engaging a multidisciplinary team, including physicians, nurses, dietitians, and pharmacists, ensures a comprehensive and collaborative approach to nutritional assessment. Each team member brings unique expertise and can contribute to a more accurate assessment and tailored nutrition plan for the patient.

5. Biochemical assessment

Alongside clinical assessments, biochemical markers can provide additional insights into the nutritional status of osteomyelitis patients. Blood tests, such as albumin, pre-albumin, and micronutrient levels, can help identify specific nutrient deficiencies or imbalances that may need to be addressed through targeted interventions.

6. Consideration of comorbidities

Osteomyelitis patients often have underlying comorbidities, such as diabetes, obesity, or cardiovascular disease, which may impact their nutritional needs. Assessing these comorbidities and their impact on nutritional status is essential for developing a comprehensive nutrition plan that addresses both the osteomyelitis and comorbidity management.

7. Monitoring and follow-up

Regular monitoring of nutritional status is crucial to evaluate the effectiveness of the nutrition plan and make necessary adjustments. Follow-up visits with the healthcare team allow for ongoing assessment, addressing any emerging challenges, and providing ongoing education and support to the patient.

8. Patient education and empowerment

Providing education to osteomyelitis patients and their caregivers about the importance of nutrition and its role in healing and recovery is vital. Empowering patients to actively participate in their nutrition care, including meal planning, food choices, and portion control, can improve adherence and overall outcomes.

9. Cultural and socioeconomic considerations

Recognizing and addressing cultural and socioeconomic factors that may impact food choices, access to nutritious foods, and dietary adherence is essential. Collaborating with the patient to develop practical and culturally sensitive dietary recommendations can enhance the success of the nutrition plan.

By addressing these barriers and challenges, healthcare professionals can conduct a comprehensive nutritional assessment for osteomyelitis patients, identify their specific nutritional needs, and develop individualized nutrition plans that optimize healing, support immune function, and promote overall well-being.

Comorbidities and nutritional needs: Tailoring dietary plans for patients with underlying conditions

When designing dietary plans for patients with underlying conditions, it's important to consider their comorbidities and individual nutritional needs. Here are some key factors to consider when tailoring dietary plans:

1. Diabetes

For patients with diabetes, managing carbohydrate intake is crucial to control blood sugar levels. Emphasize complex carbohydrates with low glycemic index, such as whole grains, legumes, and nonstarchy vegetables. Encourage portion control and regular monitoring of blood sugar levels. In some cases, coordination with a registered dietitian specializing in diabetes care may be beneficial.

2. Cardiovascular disease

For patients with cardiovascular disease, promote a heart-healthy diet that is low in saturated and trans fats, cholesterol, and sodium. Encourage consumption of lean proteins, such as fish and poultry, and incorporate sources of unsaturated fats, such as nuts, seeds, and avocados. Emphasize a variety of fruits, vegetables, whole grains, and fiber-rich foods. Limit processed and high-sugar foods.

3. Renal disease

In patients with renal disease, dietary modifications may be necessary to manage fluid and electrolyte balance, as well as protein and phosphorus intake. Depending on the severity of renal impairment, individualized recommendations for sodium, potassium, and fluid intake may be required. Collaboration with a registered dietitian specializing in renal nutrition is important to develop a suitable plan.

4. Gastrointestinal disorders

Patients with gastrointestinal disorders, such as Crohn's disease, ulcerative colitis, or irritable bowel syndrome, may require specific dietary approaches. These may include identifying trigger foods, managing fiber intake, and considering a low-FODMAP (fermentable oligosaccharides, disaccharides, monosaccharides, and polyols) diet. A registered dietitian experienced in gastrointestinal disorders can provide tailored guidance.

5. Food allergies and intolerances

Patients with food allergies or intolerances require careful assessment of their dietary needs. Identify allergens or trigger foods and work with the patient to develop a safe and balanced meal plan that avoids those foods while ensuring adequate nutrition. Consultation with a registered dietitian specializing in food allergies and intolerances may be beneficial.

6. Obesity

Obesity is a complex condition that often requires a multifaceted approach. Focus on energy balance and individualized calorie control. Encourage the consumption of nutrient-dense foods while reducing calorie-dense and processed foods. Promote portion control, mindful eating, regular physical activity, and behavior modification techniques. Collaboration with a registered dietitian specializing in weight management is recommended.

7. Cancer

Nutritional needs may vary depending on the type and stage of cancer, as well as treatment modalities. Support patients with cancer by addressing their specific symptoms, such as appetite changes, taste alterations, or difficulty swallowing. Encourage a well-balanced diet that includes lean proteins, whole grains, fruits, vegetables, and healthy fats. A registered dietitian experienced in oncology nutrition can provide tailored guidance.

Remember that each patient's situation is unique, and it's essential to consider their individual health status, preferences, cultural background, and socioeconomic factors when developing dietary plans. Collaborating with a registered dietitian or nutritionist can help ensure personalized and effective dietary recommendations that address the patient's underlying conditions and promote overall health and well-being.

Multidisciplinary Approach: Collaboration between Healthcare Professionals to address the Complex Nutritional Needs of Osteomyelitis Patients

Addressing the complex nutritional needs of osteomyelitis patients requires a multidisciplinary approach involving collaboration among healthcare professionals. By working together, healthcare providers can provide comprehensive care and optimize patient outcomes. Here are key professionals who can contribute to this multidisciplinary approach:

1. Physicians

Physicians play a central role in diagnosing and managing osteomyelitis. They assess the overall health status of the patient, prescribe appropriate medications (including antibiotics), and monitor the progress of treatment. Physicians collaborate with other healthcare professionals to ensure nutritional considerations are integrated into the overall care plan.

2. Registered Dietitians/Nutritionists

Registered dietitians or nutritionists are experts in assessing nutritional status, developing personalized nutrition plans, and educating patients on dietary modifications. They consider the specific nutritional needs of osteomyelitis patients, addressing factors such as increased nutrient requirements, potential deficiencies, and barriers to adequate food intake. Dietitians collaborate with the healthcare team to ensure patients receive optimal nutrition for healing and recovery.

3. Nurses

Nurses play a vital role in the day-to-day care of osteomyelitis patients. They monitor vital signs, administer medications, assist with wound care, and provide ongoing support. Nurses communicate with dietitians, physicians, and other healthcare professionals to ensure the nutritional aspects of care are implemented consistently and effectively.

4. Pharmacists

Pharmacists are knowledgeable about medications, including antibiotics commonly used in osteomyelitis treatment. They can provide valuable insights regarding potential interactions between medications and nutrition, such as antibiotics affecting nutrient absorption. Pharmacists collaborate with physicians and dietitians to optimize medication regimens and minimize any adverse effects on nutrition.

5. Physical Therapists/Occupational Therapists

Physical therapists and occupational therapists play a crucial role in rehabilitation and restoring functional abilities. They can assess and address any physical limitations or challenges that may impact nutrition, such as difficulty with feeding or swallowing. Collaboration with these professionals ensures that nutritional interventions are tailored to the patient's physical capabilities and promotes optimal recovery.

6. Social Workers

Social workers provide support in addressing social, emotional, and practical challenges that may affect nutrition. They can assist with accessing resources for food security, coordinating home healthcare services, and addressing any psychosocial factors that impact nutrition and overall well-being. Social workers collaborate with the healthcare team to address the holistic needs of osteomyelitis patients.

7. Occupational Therapists

Occupational therapists focus on improving the activities of daily living (ADLs) and assistive device selection for patients with osteomyelitis. They can address any limitations or difficulties in food preparation, meal planning, or feeding techniques. Collaboration with occupational therapists ensures that the patient's nutritional needs are considered within the context of their functional abilities and promotes independence in self-care.

8. Psychologists/Psychiatrists

Mental health professionals play a crucial role in supporting osteomyelitis patients who may experience emotional distress, anxiety, or depression related to their condition. These professionals can help address any psychological barriers to nutrition, such as disordered eating patterns, and provide strategies for managing stress and emotional well-being. Collaboration with mental health professionals ensures a holistic approach to patient care.

9. Speech-Language Pathologists

Speech-language pathologists can assess and address swallowing difficulties (dysphagia) that may arise in osteomyelitis patients. They provide interventions and strategies to improve swallowing function, such as modified texture diets or swallowing exercises. Collaborating with speech-language pathologists ensures that patients with dysphagia receive appropriate support and guidance for safe and effective oral intake.

10. Case Managers

Case managers play a crucial role in coordinating and managing the overall care of osteomyelitis patients. They facilitate communication among healthcare professionals, help navigate the healthcare system, and ensure continuity of care. Case managers collaborate with the multidisciplinary team to ensure that nutritional needs are addressed and incorporated into the patient's care plan.

11. Home Healthcare Providers

In cases where osteomyelitis patients receive care at home, home healthcare providers play an important role in delivering nursing care, wound care, and assisting with activities of daily living. Collaborating with home healthcare providers ensures that the nutritional aspects of care are properly implemented in the home setting and that patients receive necessary support for their nutritional needs.

Effective communication, regular interdisciplinary meetings, and shared care plans are essential for a successful multidisciplinary approach. Each professional brings their unique expertise and perspective, contributing to the holistic care of osteomyelitis patients. By working together, healthcare professionals can address the complex nutritional needs of patients, optimize nutritional support, and enhance patient outcomes and quality of life.

Patient education and compliance: Enhancing awareness and ensuring adherence to nutritional recommendations.

Patient education and ensuring adherence to nutritional recommendations are crucial aspects of managing osteomyelitis and optimizing patient outcomes.

Here are key strategies to enhance awareness and promote compliance:

1. Clear and concise communication

Healthcare professionals should provide clear and easy-to-understand information about the importance of nutrition in osteomyelitis management. Use plain language and avoid medical jargon to ensure patients comprehend the recommendations fully.

2. Individualized approach

Tailor nutritional recommendations to the patient's specific needs, preferences, and cultural background. Engage patients in discussions about their dietary habits, preferences, and challenges to develop a personalized nutrition plan that is realistic and sustainable.

3. Visual aids and written materials

Utilize visual aids, such as diagrams or illustrations, to enhance understanding of nutritional concepts. Provide written materials, such as handouts or pamphlets that summarize key points and recommendations. These resources can serve as references for patients to reinforce their understanding and adherence to nutritional guidelines.

4. Demonstration and practical guidance

Show patients how to prepare and consume recommended foods through demonstrations or videos. Offer practical guidance on meal planning, portion control, and label reading to empower patients in making informed food choices.

5. Emphasize the benefits

Educate patients on the specific benefits of proper nutrition in managing osteomyelitis. Highlight how adequate nutrition can support the healing process, boost immune function, and reduce the risk of complications. Reinforce that nutrition plays a vital role in overall health and well-being.

6. Address barriers and challenges

Identify and address potential barriers that may hinder adherence to nutritional recommendations. These barriers can include financial constraints, lack of access to healthy foods, cultural preferences, or physical limitations. Collaborate with patients to find practical solutions and alternatives that align with their circumstances.

7. Regular follow-up and support

Schedule regular follow-up appointments to monitor patients' progress, address concerns, and provide ongoing support. Utilize these opportunities to reinforce nutritional education, answer questions, and make necessary adjustments to the nutrition plan as needed.

8. Engage family and caregivers

Involve family members and caregivers in the patient's nutritional education and support. They play a crucial role in assisting with meal preparation, ensuring compliance with dietary recommendations, and providing encouragement.

9. Motivational interviewing and behavior change techniques

Employ motivational interviewing techniques to understand patients' motivations, values, and goals related to nutrition. Use behavior change techniques to facilitate positive changes in dietary habits and promote long-term adherence. Encourage patients to set realistic and achievable goals and celebrate their successes along the way.

10. Referrals and interdisciplinary collaboration

Refer patients to registered dietitians, nutritionists, or support groups specializing in nutrition education and counseling. Collaborate with these professionals to provide comprehensive and coordinated care, ensuring patients receive the necessary expertise and ongoing support for their nutritional needs.

By incorporating these strategies, healthcare professionals can enhance patient awareness, empower them to make informed choices, and promote adherence to nutritional recommendations in the management of osteomyelitis. Effective patient education and compliance can lead to improved treatment outcomes and overall well-being.

Conclusion

Optimizing nutrition plays a crucial role in the healing process and prevention of osteomyelitis. Adequate intake of essential nutrients, protein, and micronutrients can enhance bone health, support tissue repair, and boost the immune system. By incorporating nutrition as an integral part of osteomyelitis management, healthcare professionals can improve patient outcomes, reduce complications, and promote overall well-being. Further research and clinical studies are warranted to continue advancing our understanding of the intricate relationship between nutrition and osteomyelitis healing and prevention.

References

https://my.clevelandclinic.org/health/diseases/9495-osteomyelitis

https://stock.adobe.com/search/images?k=osteomyelitis

https://www.hopkinsmedicine.org/health/conditions-and-diseases/osteomyelitis

https://www.mayoclinic.org/diseases-conditions/osteomyelitis/symptoms-causes/syc-20375913

https://www.vinmec.com/vi/news/health-news/pediatrics/infectious-osteomyelitis-in-children/